Wee Small Stretch Book

KATHLEEN CONKLIN

Some small part of you wants to stretch.

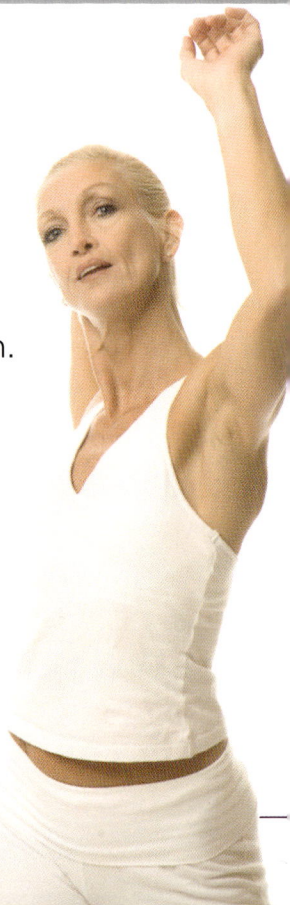

Photo Credit: Zane Williams

Wee Small Stretch Book

Preface

This book was designed in response to consistent inquiries from clients for a tool to keep up their practice of stretching safely and effectively while on the road or otherwise away from class. The human body is infinite in its possibilities for movement, though duly constrained by the Goddess Gravity and the Caliban or Peter Pan of your unique gene map. Still, there are some disciplines that survive time and science as being worthy of the catalogue of stretch techniques that consistently are safe and yet effective. Though well-researched for stretch theories and experience, this book does not purport to say or show them all. This is just the script from one stretch class – shared twice per week for 12 years.

There are risks inherent in movement programs. Changes may occur as a result of these stretch and strength practices. These include feeling tired, increased energy, mood changes, and possible short term aggravation of existing symptoms. And yet, I say I bet you will feel better.

This is a brief book. A WEE book. Not a WHY book. It shows you and tells you what to do and how to do it without getting deeply into the 'why'. Approach it as if being advised to put air in your tires and how much, without having to know the intricacies of the physical and chemical properties of the tire, the air, the gauge, or the driver. Not that you ought not know those intricacies. You are urged to learn the astounding attributes of your tires. But, this is a practice book. Any more detail will not fit into your bag lightly.

Thumbnail of the Wee Small Stretch Book Practice

The Wee Small Stretch Book Practice is a comprehensive program to stretch and support the entire body. The Practice is intended to have a flow or choreography. With patience, you will be able to transition smoothly from one stretch pattern into the next. Take your time.

Read the section titled "Stretching Essentials" to determine general rules about enhancing flexibility. Read "Master Breathing" to gain a mastery of this otherwise inevitable process. Read "Caveats" as often as needed. The entire sequence of stretches in "The Practice" which follows has a logic. Often there is not time for such full theory, though. Then follow "Can Do Today".

You will read the instruction "Inhale for a count of four and exhale for four counts and repeat three times" through the program. This is about 30 seconds of stretching. This is an excellent preparation *before* an activity, such as walking or cycling. If you are engaging in the program as an activity in its own right, consider increasing the number of breathing cycles while keeping the depth and length of each breath consistent and slow. Finally, this program works well *after* an activity to restore the muscles and quiet the breath and mind. While the longer and deeper stretches have a cumulative effect of lengthening muscles and opening joint spaces, the immediate effect is to somewhat destabilize the muscle. You do not want to do protracted stretches right before engaging in repetitive or competitive physical activity.

There are several different variations of calf, quadriceps, hip flexor and hamstrings stretches. These are not redundant. The muscles are stretched in different bone positions and in different weight-bearing positions, thus providing a more uniform stretch to each muscle through all of its actions and relationships. (You do not have to do both the Quadriceps Stretch and the Standing Quadriceps Stretch. The latter is an option in environments where you might not be able to sit down, such as the market's checkout line.)

Really, though, you are encouraged to take this as a process. A process to conscious stretching. Do not feel that you have failed if you cannot hold a stretch as long as the breathing cycles will ask of you. You have not failed if you cannot hold your arms in the air for very long. Pick three stretches to start. Choose those you like. It is okay to like this work and to like moving your body and to feel good moving. Practice those three for ten days. Pick three others. You can choose any three but you don't have to choose what order to do them in; just follow the sequence in the Practice. Ritual should make you conscious, not bored.

And yet, do not hold back. Do more if you are excited about it or even intrigued. Your body knows when to stop and when to get more and it loves this work. Listen to your body. Look in. Connect the dots. What is the same about the three stretches you picked? What are differences? Why did you wait on the others? Nothing changes without conscious attention to the choice.

Finally, don't look at the body in this book as a goal. Look at it like a live drawing. Like the depiction of enjoyment of moving, an illustration of one body in motion, a logic showing the relationship of the literal instructions to the bone rhythms in your own body. Enjoy your own dialect of this body language.

TABLE OF CONTENTS

STRETCHING ESSENTIALS   1-4
Let's put a little "zing" into your human movement potential.

MASTER BREATHING   5-10
Breathing goes to your head.

CAVEATS   11-12
Ways to play it safe.

THE PRACTICE
The full program is intended to have a flow or choreography to it. With a bit of practice, you will be able to transition smoothly from one stretch pattern into the next.

Neutral Body Posture	13-14
Full Body Upstretch	15-16
Torso Side Stretch	17-18
Jazz Hands and Arms Stretch	19-20
Calf to Hamstrings Series	21-28
Standing Calf Stretch	23-24
Long Bridge Calf Stretch	25-26
Standing Hamstrings Stretch	27-28

Quad/Hip/Hamstrings series-	29-40
Deep Lunge, Parallel	31-32
Deep Lunge, Rotated	33-34
Hamstrings, Parallel	35-36
Hamstrings, Rotated	37-38
Hurdle Stretch	39-40
Quadriceps Stretch	41-42
Standing Quadriceps Stretch	43-44
Sides of Buttocks and Thighs	45-46
External Rotators Stretch	47-48
Inner Thigh Stretch	49-50
Neck Stretch	51-52
Foot/Ankle	53-54
Abdominal Curls	55-56
CAN DO TODAY	57-58
THE FULL PRACTICE IN PICTURES	59-60
BIOGRAPHY	61
ACKNOWLEDGEMENTS	62

STRETCHING ESSENTIALS

Let's put a little "zing" into your human movement potential. Stretching helps you move, helps you breathe, helps you be.

Essentials of moving

- One side lengthens for the opposing side to shorten.
- One side of the body expands for the opposing side to contract.
- One side of the body, then, stretches, for the opposing side to strengthen.
- Stretch is necessary to being able to move, stretch is essential to moving with ease.

Stop thinking stretching is a waste of time. You absolutely could not move if muscles did not 'stretch.'

You have to stretch because you have to. All locomotion, even the tiniest movement, requires one group of muscles to lengthen, or stretch, in order for the opposing muscle or muscle group to contract and thereby move the levers of your bones to move you. Those rhythms happen naturally in the architecture of our bodies. But, if you stretch consciously, knowingly, you optimize the power inherent in that blueprint and minimize the drag on your system which creates inefficiencies and fatigue.

Gateways to flexibility

Warm muscles stretch farther and with more ease. Muscles may be warmed in water, air or by moving. A sauna, or hot bath can warm muscles sufficiently to enhance stretch. Be cautious, though, extremely hot conditions can confuse signals in the body so that you may be stretching connective tissue, nerves or joints, rather than muscle. Activities where you use the body more than passively will also warm the muscles. The order of this Practice gets you moving and warming and then moves into the more intense stretches. You can also do these stretches after other activities like sports or games, and after repetitive motion like walking or running.

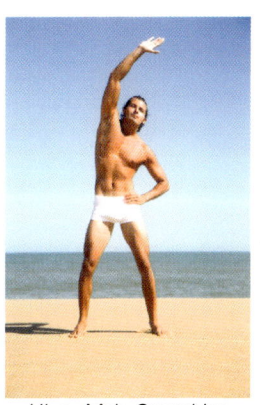

Uhm. Male Stretching

Muscle stretches enhance flexibility in movement and range of motion. Stretching the joints can be destabilizing and permanent. Feeling pain at a joint is not indicative of muscle stretching. Stretching muscles to the threshold of stoicism is counter-productive. A stretch that is too intense will trigger the opposite response in the muscle. The muscle spindles in the belly of the muscle will indicate it is stretching too far too

Stretching Essentials

fast and cause a contraction. This is not producing a flexible muscle. Hold a stretch at the threshold where it is pleasantly uncomfortable and you can still breathe.

Holding a stretch long enough for the nervous system to recognize that the muscle is allowed to stop contracting will facilitate flexibility and new length in muscle fibers. Most of these stretches are held statically for 30 seconds. A shorter stretch is probably not worth the time – there is no new information for the nervous system to incorporate. Longer stretches do provide new neuromuscular information and lengthening, but they can be temporarily destabilizing. So don't hold a stretch for four minutes and then go out for a six mile run.

Sequencing

Studies show that stretching muscles in a certain order can enhance flexibility. Stretching one group of muscles before another will ease and facilitate the stretch of the next group. Examples:

- Calves before Hamstrings
- Quadriceps before Sides of Buttocks and Thighs

- Quadriceps before Inner Thighs
- Superficial muscles to Deep muscles

Cues and other Assists

In this Stretch Practice, look for and consider the following cues to make each stretch safe, more effective, more efficient, more powerful.

- Alignment cue
- Breath cue
- Safety cue
- Intensity cue
- Imagery or visualization cue

Master Breathing

- 26,000 times per day, or more, you breathe

- Ventilation (breathing) is non-negotiable but subject to mastery

- Breathing oscillates the spine and spine oscillation is an internal massage

- Breathe into your back

- Breathe to a count, don't hold the breath

- Deep breathing both requires abdominal muscle strength and creates it

- Breathing through your nose goes to your head

There are three parts to the breathing cycle, *exhalation, pause, inhalation.* The pause is that moment of rest while the body collects itself to work the inhale and then work the exhale.

Lie down for a moment (knees bent up, feet flat, legs parallel) and notice your breathing.

The diaphragm is the primary breathing muscle. It moves the chest cavity and changes its volume in three directions, up and down, side to side, and front to back. It does 70-80% of the work of quiet breathing. One of its attachments is on the front of the spine inside your body. When the diaphragm moves up and down, it gently pulls on the spine, creating an oscillation. On an inhale, the spine typically comes up off of the floor. On the exhale, the spine settles down.

Everyone's quiet breathing pattern is different. Like a fingerprint or signature. Notice if your spine moves a lot or a little as you inhale and exhale. This oscillation of the spine is a brilliant mechanism in the body for keeping the discs between the vertebrae supple, and for assisting the spinal fluid circulation and supporting its pulse. Spine oscillation is an internal massage.

Do you notice the *pause* in your breathing cycle? You use the breathing muscles 22-26,000 times per day. They like that moment of quiet between exhaling and inhaling.

Inhalation and exhalation, also referred to as inspiration and expiration, are the respiration or breathing cycle. Healthy people use additional muscles to force inhalation and increase both the rate and volume of air intake in exercise.

Master Breathing

Forced Inhalation Forced inspiration – consider that you are being inspired with every new breath. Many of the muscles used to aggressively inhale are in your *back*. Six muscle groups are in, or start in, your back to help hold the rib case out to help the diaphragm create more volume. At the greatest inhalation, you can breathe down to your 11th rib on the right and your 12th rib on the left. That is, you can if the muscles are flexible enough and strong enough to allow the rib case to expand in the first place. If you breathe that deeply, you are drawing breath to the lowest lobes of your lungs. The right lung has three lobes, the left has two to make room for the heart. The lowest lobes of your lungs are highly vascularized. In other words, they get the most blood flow. If you get more air to the bottom of your lungs, you get more enriching oxygen to your bloodstream faster and with less demand on the heart. More oxygen to your bloodstream gets more to your muscles faster too.

Breathing through your nose is better. Breathing through your nose humidifies, warms and cleans the air you breathe. If for no other reason, breathe clean, warm moist air into the miraculous organs that are your lungs.

There is another reason. Breathing through the nose facilitates the parasympathetic nervous system. This is the system that keeps you functioning while you are consciously attending to other things. In the alternative, breathing through your mouth can stimulate the sympathetic nervous system, commonly referred to as the fight or flight response system. Breathing through the nose signals the body to associate moving and breathing and stretching with calmness, serenity and intention without anxiety. That, in turn, conditions you to be able to respond in other situations with calm, serenity and intention.

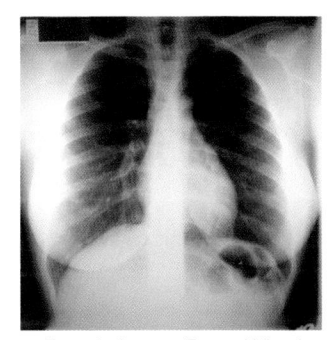

Female Lungs (Frontal View)

- Breathe into your back. Visualize your lungs moving down to the base of your ribs. Think of breathing into the soft tissue of your back.

- Breathe through your nose.

Do you ever feel like you can't catch your breath or get enough? Do you inhale more? The air is likely getting only to the top lobes of the lungs which are not as efficient at exchanging oxygen and carbon dioxide. Try exhaling first. Empty every bit of air from the lungs.

Master Breathing

Forced Exhalation Expiration – a short death from which you are inspired to breathe again. Do it now. Exhale.

Keep exhaling. Are you still?

During quiet breathing, the diaphragm moves up toward your head to exhale the lungs. The diaphragm pulls down toward your feet to inhale the lungs. The pelvic floor muscles move in the same direction, or parallel with the diaphragm. The pelvic floor muscles are slung from your pubic bones to tail bones and sitbones. They open and close for reproduction and elimination activities. And they release and contract to support the organs and the diaphragm in breathing. Practice closing the pelvic floor muscles to each other. Imagine stopping the urine flow mid-stream, then release, then repeat. The contraction-release of the pelvic floor muscles affects all of the body's systems, as well as your elegance in moving.

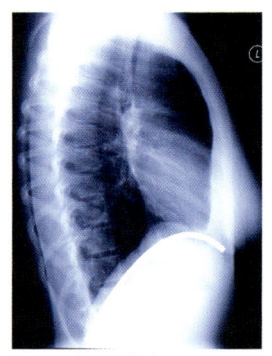

*Female Lungs
Lateral View (Side)
The diaphragm muscle is the line between the white space in the belly and the dark of the lungs above. The line of the muscle travels from the mid-front of the body up, and then down the slope to the lower back ribs.*

Exhale for 16 counts. The infamous abs. Besides the pelvic floor, you need the four abdominal muscles to aggressively exhale. Transversus, the muscle that runs around the waist like a wide belt, is the deepest. It compresses the guts when it contracts. This increased pressure pushes the diaphragm up forcefully which helps squeeze air out of the lungs. So belly muscles help you exhale.

Exhale through the nose. Because the airway is smaller, you need more support to move the air out of the body fast enough. Exhaling through the nose creates a greater demand on the abdominals and other muscles which facilitate breathing. Really, though, abdominal muscles are not just powerful exhalers, they also enhance the inhale. The more the diaphragm gets stretched up on exhale, the greater its rebound or contraction (or counter-action) for the next inhale. Strong abdominal muscles get you more volume, more fuel, more power, less strain in breathing.

- Breathing is at the medulla oblongata in your brain. It will happen anyway but you can drive it. A deep exhale triggers instinctual inhale.

- Strengthen your abdominal muscles to improve your breathing.

Caveats

- IF IT HURTS, STOP. Stretching should not hurt at a joint. Useful and efficient stretch can feel good. At the level where it is increasing suppleness of muscle, it can be uncomfortable. But stretching should never require stoicism. That is actually counter-productive.

- Notice if you are holding your breath. Exhale. If you are not breathing, you cannot be stretching. The body will be held too rigidly.

- Be in the stretch where it is substantially uncomfortable but not in searing or specific pain.

- Being in the stretch means being alive in it, not stuck in it or rigid.

- Do not bob up and down in a stretch, deepen the stretch on each breath.

- *Before* an activity, be in the stretch about 30 seconds. Better yet, 'count' the stretch with breathwork, inhaling for four counts, exhaling for four counts, three to five times.

- *After* an activity, stretching should take a minute or more for each single muscle or small group of muscles. Better yet, 'count' the stretch with breathwork, inhaling for four counts, exhaling for six to eight counts about eight times.

- Remember, inhaling is breathing into your back, exhaling is pressing all of the air out with your pelvic floor and abdominals. Breathing in and out through your nose facilitates your parasympathetic nervous system, the part of the system that is usually not consciously controlled and which slows you into at-rest mode or serene functioning.

- Cramps? Lift your big toe, it will contract a muscle group opposing the action of the one or more muscles cramping (a non-smooth muscle contraction) or it will just sufficiently distract you so that the cramp subsides…

Not Neutral but a good chest expansion stretch

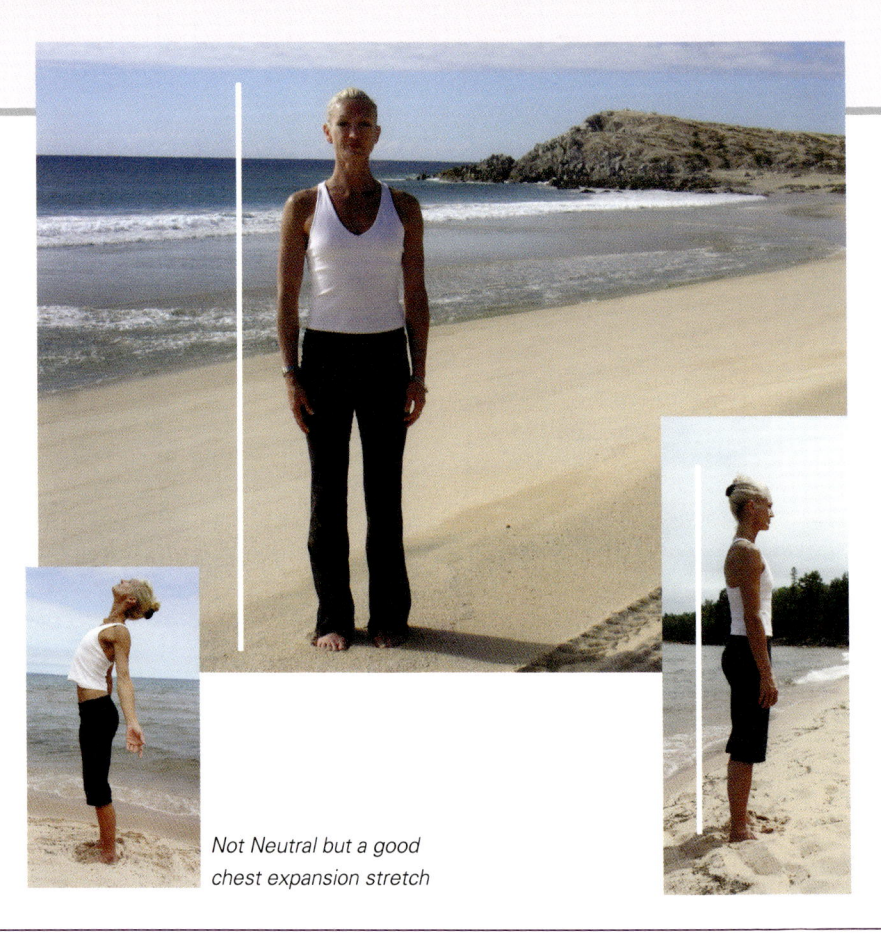

Neutral Body Posture

Stand, feet parallel to each other. The second toe, next to the big toe, should be in line with the center of the heel. The heels and second toes should be the same distance apart. Line up the legs parallel with each other directly under the femoral joint (hips). The femoral joint is about halfway between your hipbone (anterior superior iliac spine, or ASIS) and your pubic bone. So the middle of the kneecap (patella) and the second toe will be in line with that joint, or halfway between hipbone and pubic bone.

Soften the knees so the kneecaps are lined up over the second toe.

Keep your pelvis neutral as you bend your knees. Do not let your sitbones (ischial tuberosities, the bones you sit on) sneak forward. The pelvis is neutral when the two hipbones are lined up with, and in the same plane as, the pubic bones. (There are two pubic bones, they are conjoined with a symphysis, or cartilage joint.)

Rib case balances over the pelvic bowl.

Skull balances over the rib case.

Ears, shoulders, femoral joints and ankles fall in the plumb-line from ceiling to floor.

Arms hang from shoulders. Hands are slightly ahead of side of thigh.

Arms, legs and spine are vertical awareness.

Ears, shoulders, hips, knees and ankles are horizontal awareness.

Correct Posture

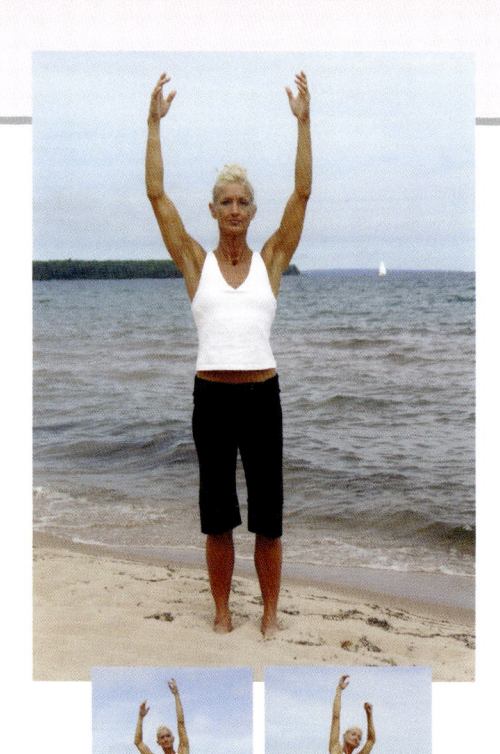

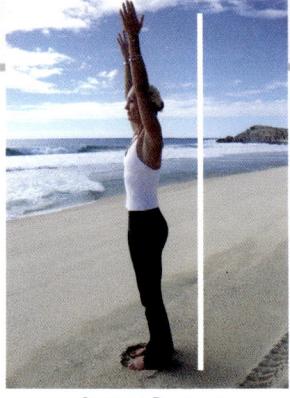

Incorrect Posture

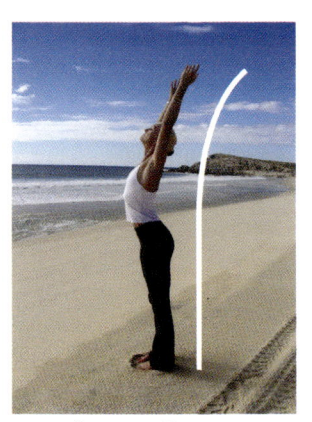

Full Body Upstretch

From **Neutral Body Posture,** reach arms upward and parallel to each other. Think of the arms sliding in vertical paths down your back to your heels.

Reach the heel of the left hand to the sky and heel of left foot to the ground. Stretch the entire left side of the body. Breathe into the left ribs. Breathe into the left lung. Stay on the flat of the left foot, though the right heel may be lifted.

Increase the intensity by reaching the heel of the hand and heel of foot away from each other. Imagine lifting the ceiling higher and pushing the floor into the planet.

Inhale into your back-ribs and the soft tissue of your back body for a count of four. Exhale for four counts, noticing your belly flatten from the inside. Feel the insides of the ribs opening on the inhale and keep them open on the exhale. Feel the left side of the body lengthen on the inhale and release on the exhale.

The four count inhale followed by the four count exhale is one full breath cycle. Be in the stretch for three full breath cycles.

Rise up on the balls of both feet. Reach heel of the right hand to the sky and heel of right foot to the ground. Repeat the breath cycles and imagery on this right side.

Repeat both sides, but start up to the right first and then stretch to the left.

To the Right

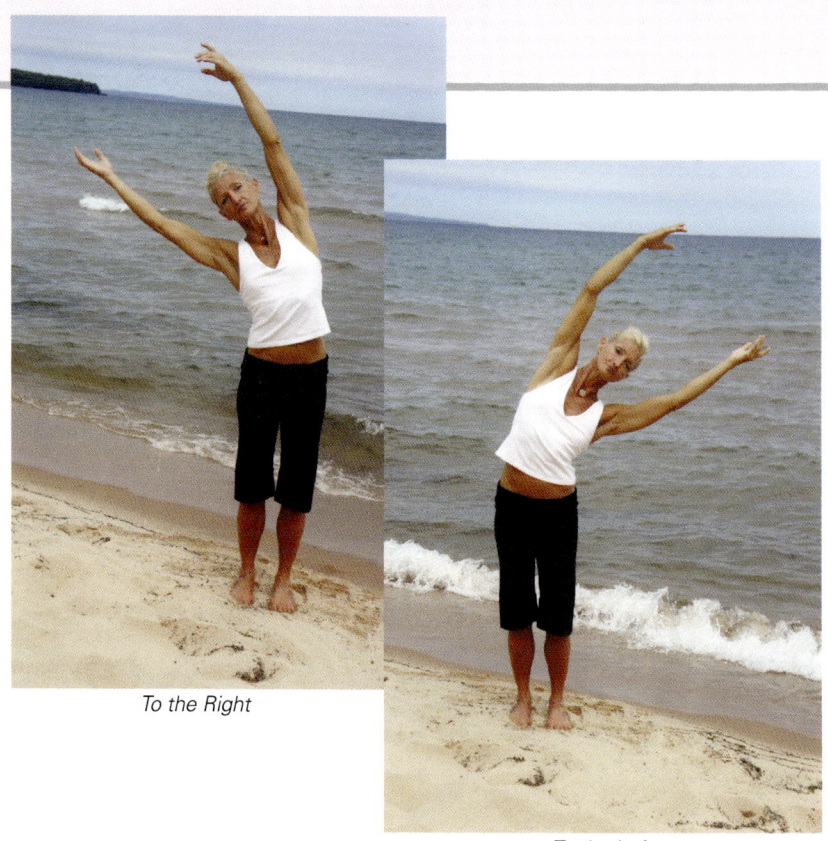

To the Left

Torso Side Stretch

From **Full Body Upstretch** flex, or bend, the knees a bit more than just a softened position. Flex, or bend, your spine to the left, meaning the head end of your spine points to the left; the spine convexes to the right. Arms stay parallel to each other, head stays evenly spaced between the arms. Pelvis stays neutral and still. Legs stay parallel, still and flexed. Imagine you are sliding sideways along a vertical wall, keeping head, shoulders, low ribs and the rest of your backside against the wall.

Inhale for four counts to flex, exhale for four counts to return to vertical. Keep spine safe by holding belly muscles in. Keep your neck safe by keeping shoulders down away from your ears. Intensify the stretch by pressing both heels into the floor (but do not lift the balls of the feet). As you flex to one side, imagine pressing the top of your head, the point on which your head would rotate on a vertical axis, out through the space between your hands.

As you flex to the left, feel the right side of the body lengthen and feel the left side stay open, uncollapsed. Feel the right side contract as you recover vertical. Think of the right rib case and right hipbone coming toward each other to recover.

Repeat the imagery and breath cycles above to the right, alternating side to side eight times.

19 Wee Small Stretch Book

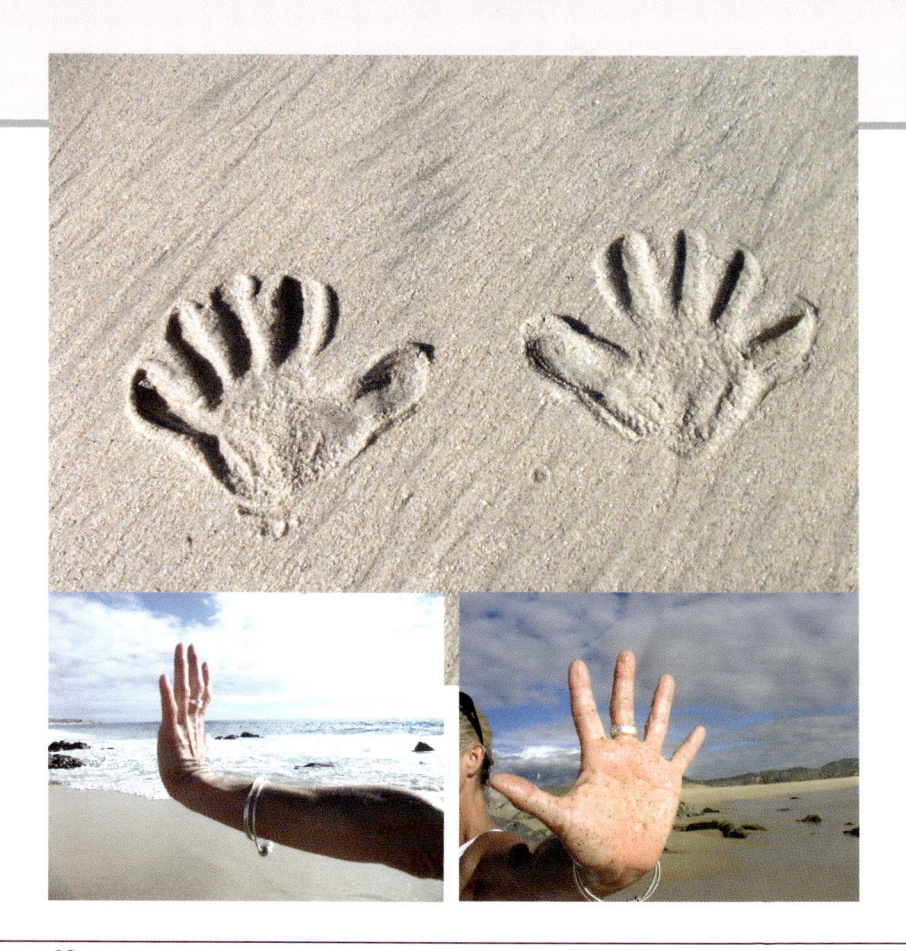

Jazz Hands and Arms Stretch

From **Torso Side Stretch** in the vertical position, unbend the knees just until they are unlocked. Open the fingers of each hand as wide as possible, arms straight overhead, palms forward. Bend the elbows, pulling hands down from vertical and press the palms of the hands out away from the sides of your body. Keep the elbows safe by not locking them. Keep the hands slightly ahead of and below the shoulder joints. Release the trapezius muscles which join your shoulders up to your neck, and thereby lower the shoulders. Intensify the stretch by pressing the heel of the hand farther away from your body than the tips of your fingers.

Imagine pressing the walls of the world away from you. Breathe into the stretch. Feel the stretch in the hands, forearms and shoulder girdle. Breathe the inhale/exhale cycle of four counts each, one to three times, whatever you can stand.

Next, rotate the arms so that the fingertips now point behind you, palms out. Repeat breathing cycles. See or feel your arms lengthening away from your collar bones.

Finally, rotate the fingertips until they point directly to the ground. Breathe the four-count cycles three times. Go for a sense of constant internal movement and lengthening rather than rigidly holding the position.

Gently shake the arms after the stretches.

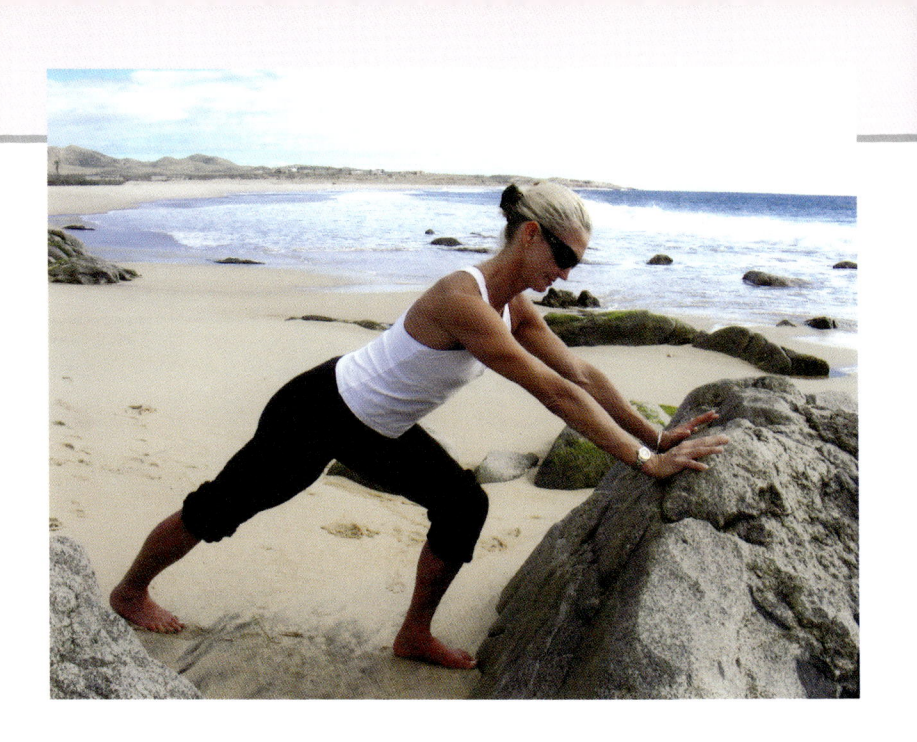

Calf to Hamstrings Series

    Standing Calf Stretch

    Long Bridge Calf Stretch

    Standing Hamstrings Stretch

This is a sequence of three stretches that follow the principle of "calves before hamstrings" as a gateway to increased flexibility in the legs. The book illustrates each stretch individually.

If your gastrocnemius and soleus muscles (the calf muscles) are tight, you might feel pain behind the knees in the calf stretches. You might also feel pain in stretching the semimembrinosis, semitendinosis, and biceps femoris. These are commonly called hamstrings, the back of the thigh.

Pelvis and rib case and head will be aligned as in the **Neutral Body Posture** (p, 14).

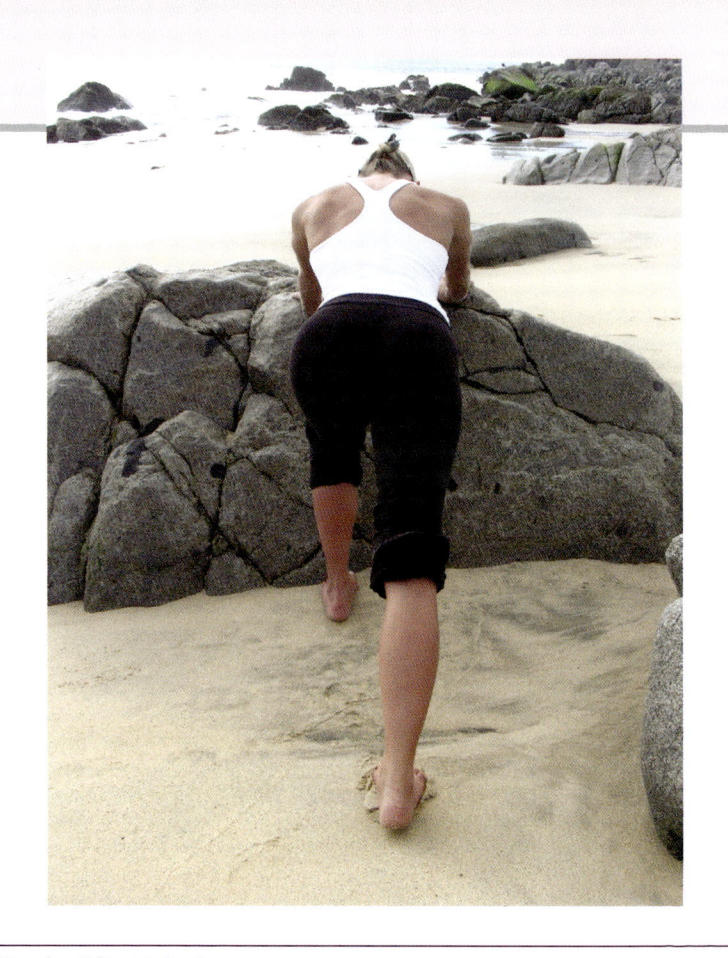

Standing Calf Stretch

Face a wall, or fence or rock, in **Neutral Body Posture.** Bring hands up to shoulder height and press hands into the wall. Reach the right foot back as you flex, bend, the left knee directly over your second toe. The center of the back of the heel should be lined up behind the ankle and with the second toe.

Inhale for a count of four and exhale for four counts and repeat three times. Inhale into the stretch, feel the release on the exhale. Intensify the stretch by pressing into the wall. Feel the heel lengthen into the floor. Keep knees over second toes and unlocked. Keep pelvis pressed forward and neutral (hipbones stay in line with each other parallel to the wall).

Repeat with the left leg back.

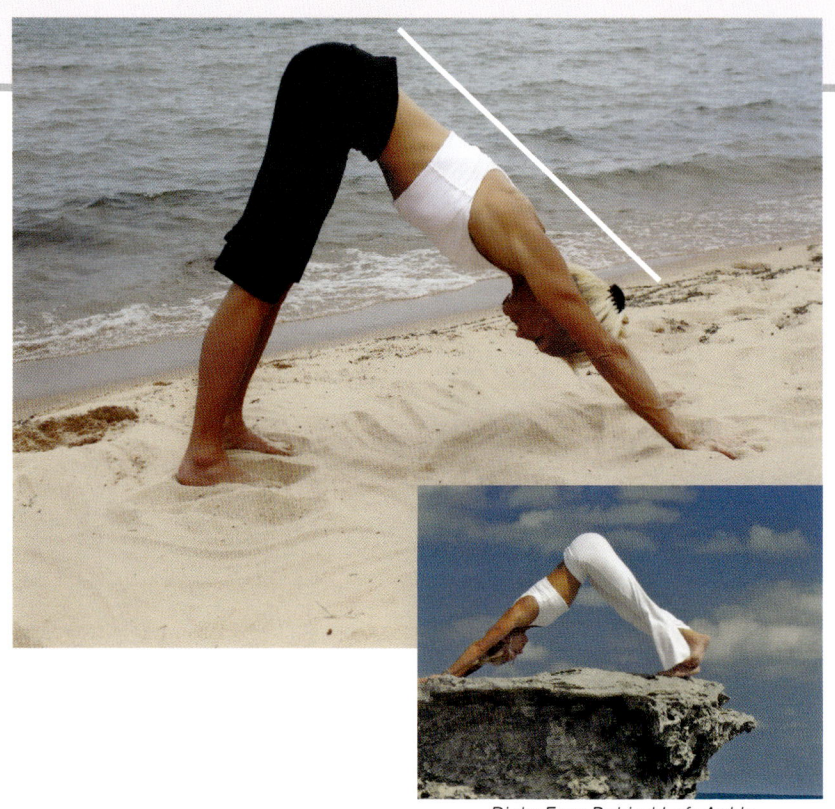

Right Foot Behind Left Ankle

LONG BRIDGE CALF STRETCH

Feet are parallel to each other and lined up under the hips (femoral joints are half way between the hipbones, or ASIS, and the pubic bone). Place hands on the ground in similar alignment to the feet and stretch sitbones up to the sky. Keep the back flat and shoulders out of the ears. Unbend the knees but do not lock them. Place right foot behind the left ankle.

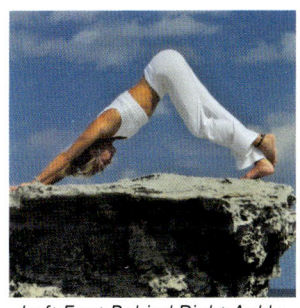

Left Foot Behind Right Ankle

Intensify the stretch in the left ankle by first pressing the heel into the ground. If you need more stretch, assist with the right foot gently pressing the left heel down. The left knee should be lined up over the second toe (next to the big toe) on the left foot. Pull the sitbones to the sky for more stretch. Keep the hipbones parallel with each other. Inhale for a count of four and exhale for four counts and repeat three times. This is a fabulous opportunity to think about breathing into and expanding the soft tissue of the back between the ribs and pelvis. Repeat with the right foot down and right calf stretching.

27 Wee Small Stretch Book

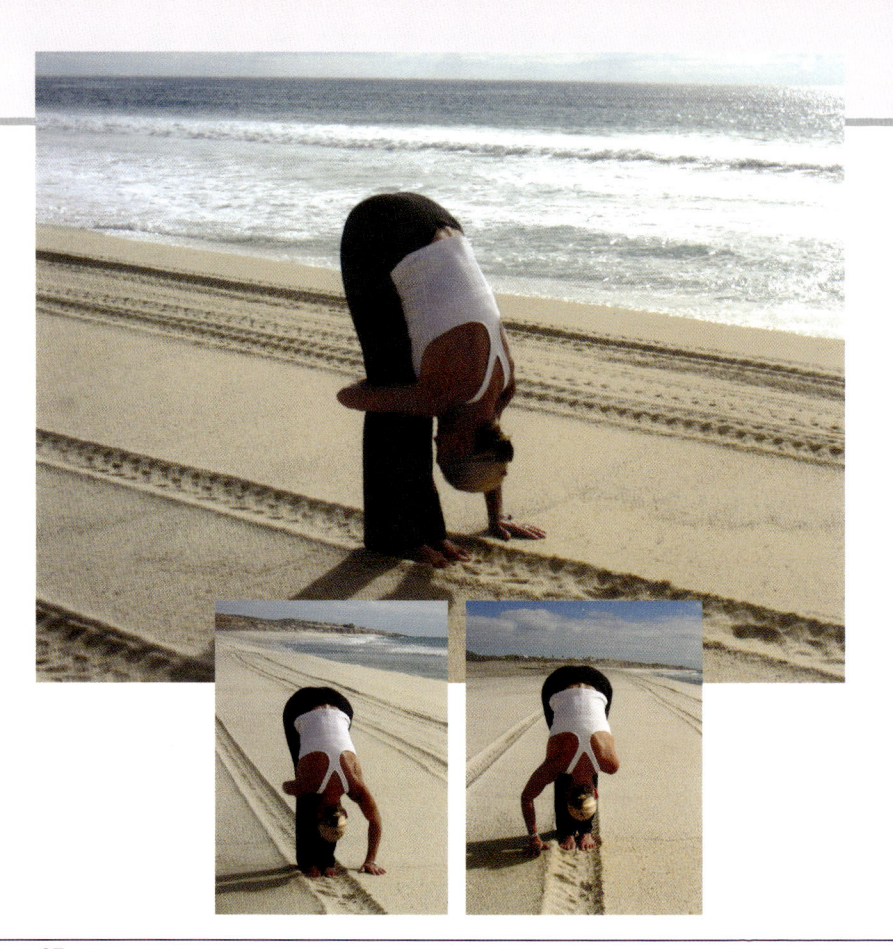

STANDING HAMSTRINGS STRETCH

From the **Long Bridge Calf Stretch,** walk your hands back toward your feet. Wrap your arms around your legs and hug your chest to your thighbones. Let the head hang. This creates traction along the spine and relieves unnecessary tension in the neck and shoulders. Gently lift both sitbones to the sky. Breathe. Do not lock the knees. Increase the stretch by lifting the sitbones higher. Let the head hang. Notice your breath. You are breathing upside down which completely changes the forces of gravity on the diaphragm and on the muscles which assist inhalation and exhalation. Inhale for a count of four and exhale for four counts and repeat three times.

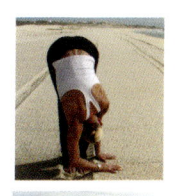

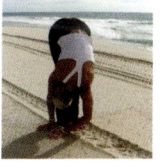

Got time? Bend the left knee and straighten the right slightly; this should give more stretch to the right hamstrings. Try to keep the hipbones level and your back long, if not flat. Inhale for a count of four and exhale for four counts and repeat three times. Switch by bending the right knee and straightening the left.

Got more time? Put both hands to the left of the left foot. Try to keep the hipbones level and your back long, if not flat. You'll feel stretch on the right torso as well. Inhale for a count of four and exhale for four counts and repeat three times. Switch by sweeping the hands to the outside of the right foot and feel the stretch on the left torso, and left hamstrings.

(Remember, pain behind knees in calf stretches or hamstrings stretches indicates you need more calf stretch.)

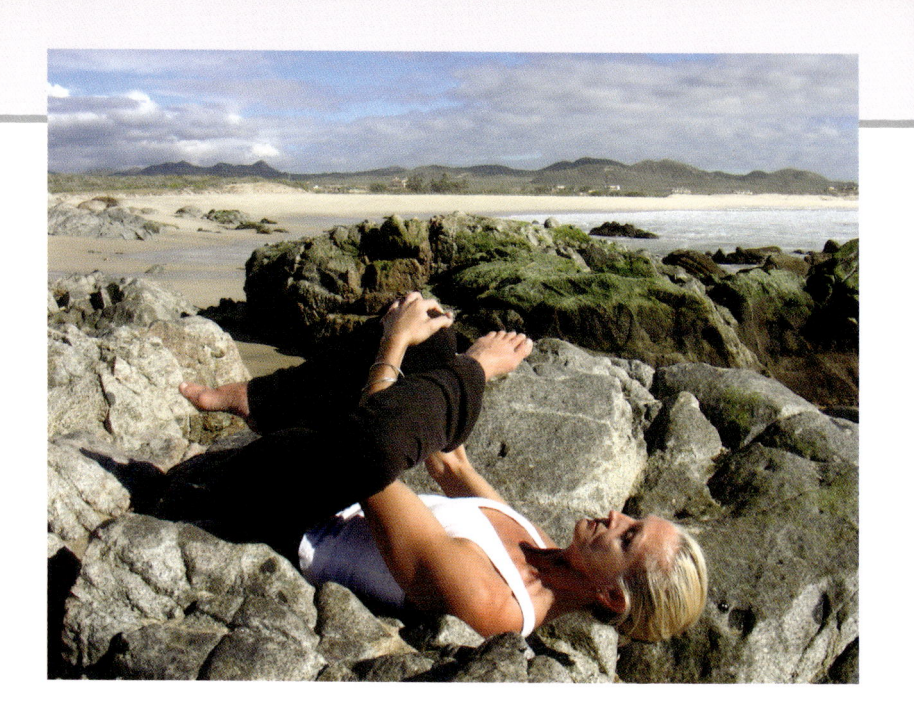

Quad/Hip/Hamstrings Series

Deep Lunge, Parallel

Deep Lunge, Rotated

Hamstrings, Parallel

Hamstrings, Rotated

Hurdle Stretch

This is a series of five stretches that flow one into the other. **Complete the series on one side of the body first; transition smoothly to the series on the other side of the body.** The book illustrates each stretch individually.

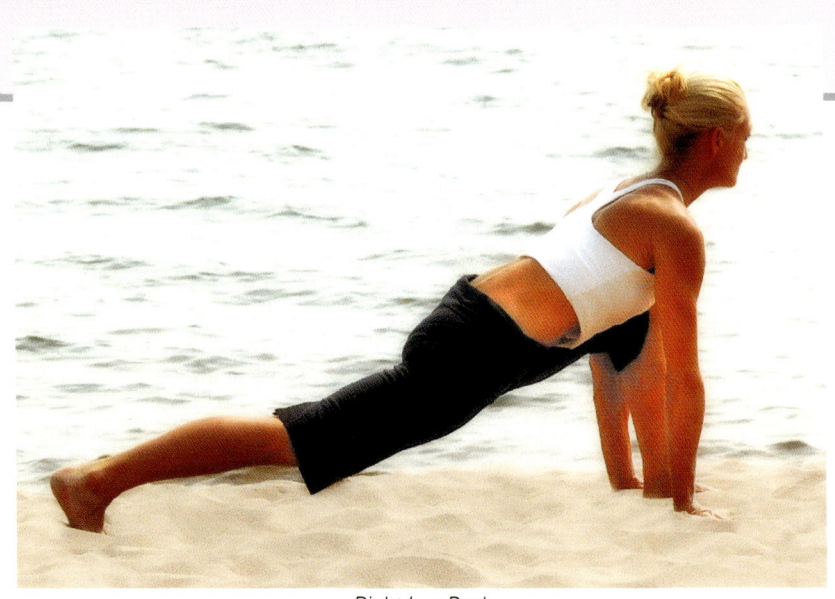

Right Leg Back

Deep Lunge, Parallel

From the **Standing Hamstrings Stretch,** slowly reach hands forward along the ground and bring one leg forward between the arms into a deep lunge. The ankle of the forward foot should be exactly under the forward knee so the knee is not over-flexed. The shin is vertical. If you cannot reach the ground with your hands, support your hands on blocks or some other sturdy structure. Both legs remain parallel. That is, the kneecap of the back leg is aiming straight at the ground and the knee of the bent leg is directly over the second toe.

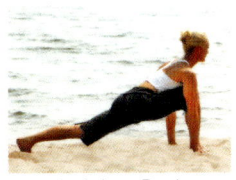

Left Leg Back

The primary stretch is in the quadriceps and hip flexor of the back leg. You might also feel stretch in the hamstrings of the forward leg. Keep the hipbones level with each other and parallel to your shoulders. Keep the flexed forward knee over the second toe and the straight knee behind you unlocked.

To intensify the stretch, squeeze the buttock of the leg that is straight back. Do not squeeze the butt under, but together to the other buttock and think of pulling the hipbone to the ribs. Press the entire pelvis forward toward the front foot. Imagine the leg lengthening out forever behind you. Let the back leg feel like mercury, running across the floor.

Do not let your head hang toward the ground. Pull the top points of your ears to up to the sky. Inhale for a count of four and exhale for four counts and repeat three times.

Transition into the next stretch, the **Deep Lunge, Rotated.**

Right Leg, Rotated

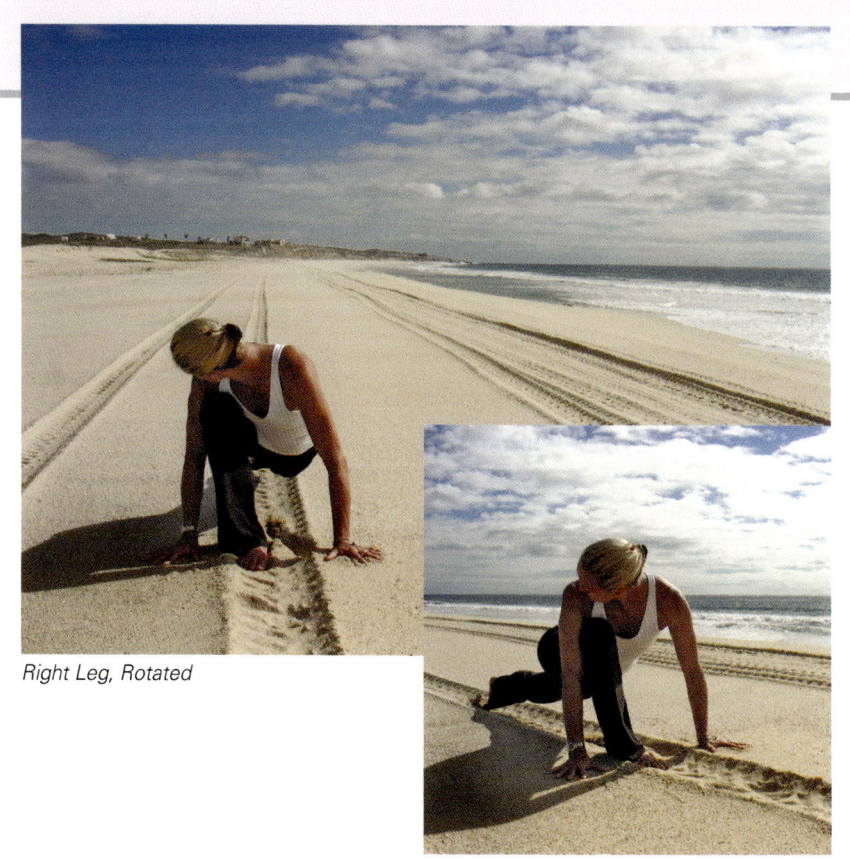

Angled View

Deep Lunge, Rotated

From the **Deep Lunge, Parallel** position, rotate your chest toward your forward leg, and allow the hip of the back leg to drop a bit toward the ground. Shift the weight to the outside of the back leg, rather than directly on top. The leg turns inward slightly. This will move the primary stretch to the outside of the hip flexor and the more lateral quadriceps muscle. It may add a bit of stretch to the latissimus dorsi and oblique muscles felt along the side of the torso stretching toward the ground.

You may feel stretch in the quadratus lumborum located between the bottom of the rib case and the top of the pelvis alongside the spine as it curves slightly toward the ground. Try to keep the forward knee from swinging outward, away from center.

Intensify the stretch, press the long back leg slightly into the ground. Imagine lengthening the back leg out forever. Keep your ears back and the crown of the head, not your face, pulling to the sky. Inhale for a count of four and exhale four counts and repeat three times.

Transition into the next stretch, **Hamstrings, Parallel.**

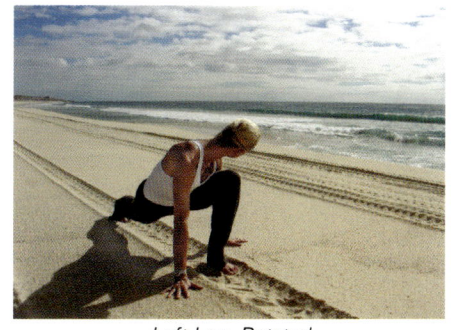

Left Leg, Rotated

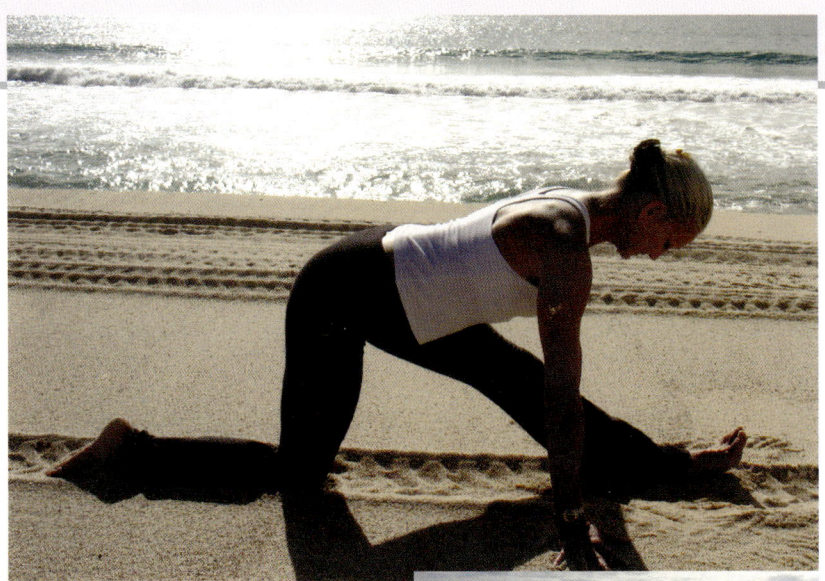

Left Leg

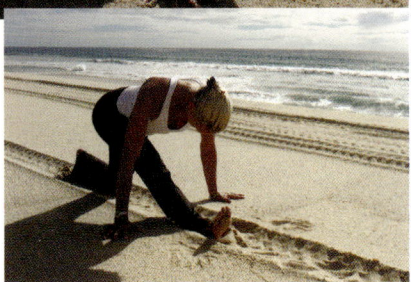

Right Leg

35 Wee Small Stretch Book

Hamstrings, Parallel

From the **Deep Lunge, Rotated** position, unrotate the torso, shift your weight back over the knee of the back leg. As you bend the back leg, straighten the forward leg. Now the primary stretch shifts to the underside of the front leg, the hamstrings.

Keep the hips and shoulders parallel. Think of squaring them with each other. Keep the weight over the supporting knee, not behind or in front of the knee. In other words, the thighbone (femur) is vertical. If you cannot reach the ground with your palms or knuckles, use blocks or other symmetrical supports on the ground under your hands for balance. To keep the stretch out of your back, and singularly in the hamstrings, try to flatten the back.

Intensify the stretch by pulling the forward foot up toward the knee, that is, dorsiflex the ankle. To further intensify the stretch as you feel the muscles begin to lengthen, pull the sitbone of the forward leg away from the heel. Breathe into the stretch. Breathe into the bones and muscles of your back. Feel the muscles release. Think of the muscles being warm. Inhale for a count of four and exhale for four counts and repeat three times.

Transition into the next stretch, **Hamstrings, Rotated.**

Anterior (Front) View

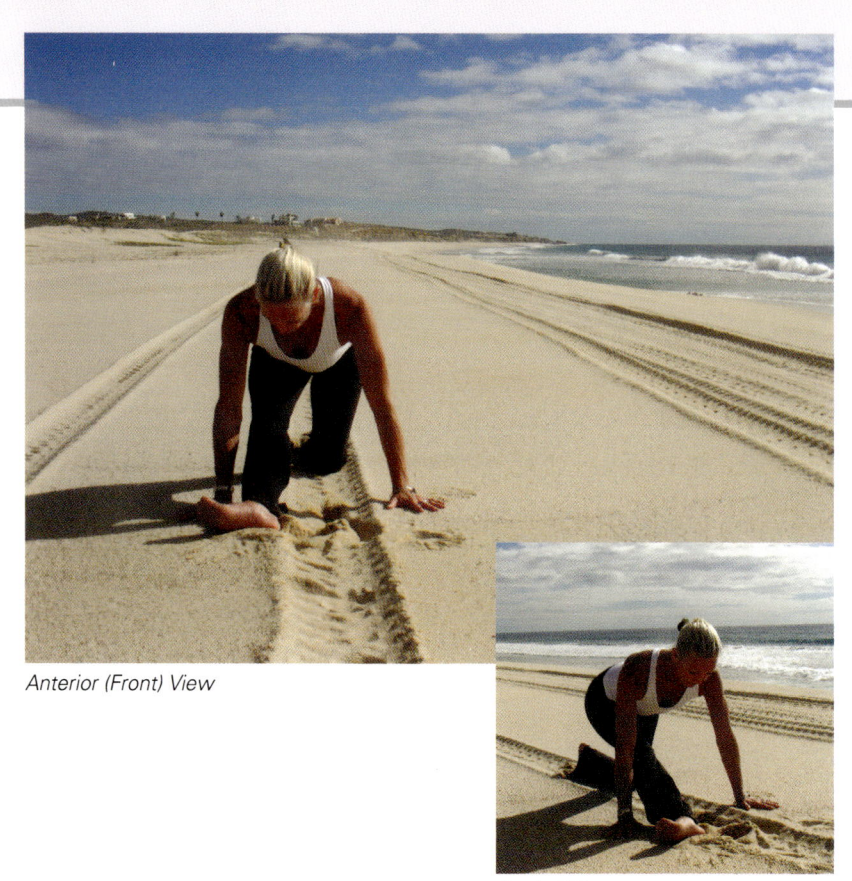

Angled View

Hamstrings, Rotated

From the **Hamstrings, Parallel** stretch, turn the forward leg in external rotation so that the outside edge of your foot is on the ground or near. Try to keep the dorsiflexion of the ankle that you created in the prior stretch position - the top of the foot pulling toward the knee. The whole forward leg is laterally rotated, turned outward from the hip (femoral joint).

This may take your breath away. Don't let it. Breathe. Inhale for a count of four and exhale for four counts and repeat breath cycle at least three times. Most people feel lateral hamstrings stretching, these are at the back but toward the side of the leg. Some will feel IT Band (iliotibial band) stretch on the side of the thigh. Keep the hips (femoral joints) level and breathe, breathe, breathe.

Transition into the next stretch, **Hurdle Stretch.**

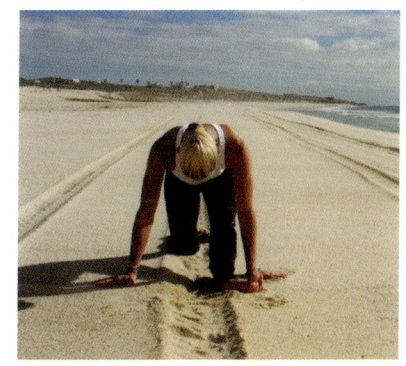

Left Leg, Rotated

Angled View

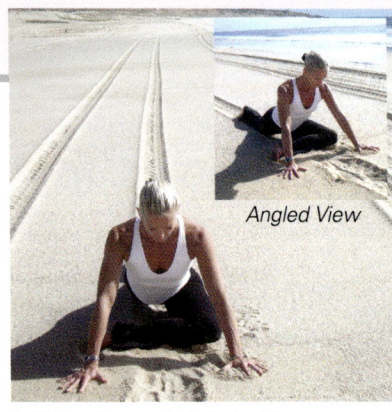

Angled View

Left Leg Forward, Anterior View

Right Leg Forward, Anterior View

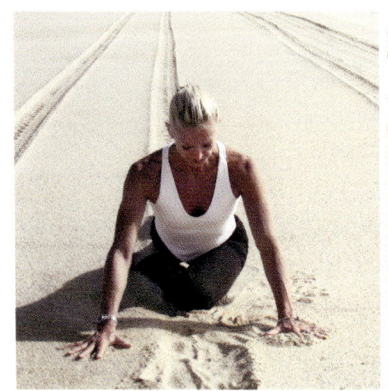

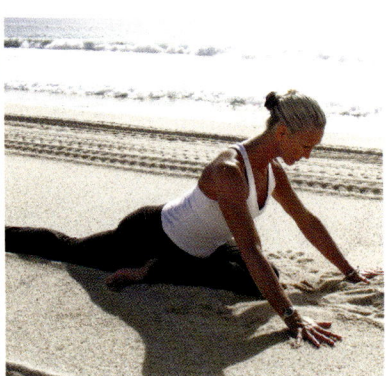

Deeper Piriformis, Knee Moved to Center of Pelvis

39 Wee Small Stretch Book

Hurdle Stretch

From the **Hamstrings, Rotated** stretch, shift your weight forward. "Walk" the forward foot sideways and back to the groin. Set your weight down on the outside of the forward leg which is fairly deeply flexed. The back leg is parallel behind you, kneecap down.

Rest your torso over the front, bent knee. You can rest your torso on the leg and the ground, or support yourself on forearms or hands. As you get more flexible, you can move the forward knee such that the forward foot comes farther away from the groin and more in line with the line of the back leg. This stretches the gluteals and the external rotators deep to the gluteals. If the forward knee is more centered with the pubic bone and the sacrum is not tucked, the stretch will be more localized in the dreaded and powerful piriformis. BREATHE. Inhale for a count of four and exhale for four counts and repeat SIX times. This is deep muscle and a lot of it. Take your time allowing all of the muscles to settle into length.

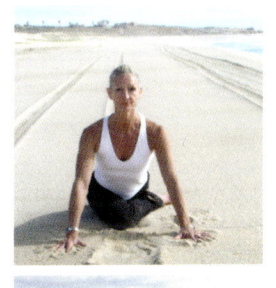

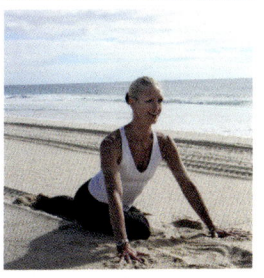

Pull the forward leg back under you and come up on both knees to start the **Quad/Hip/Hamstrings Series** again with the other leg forward.

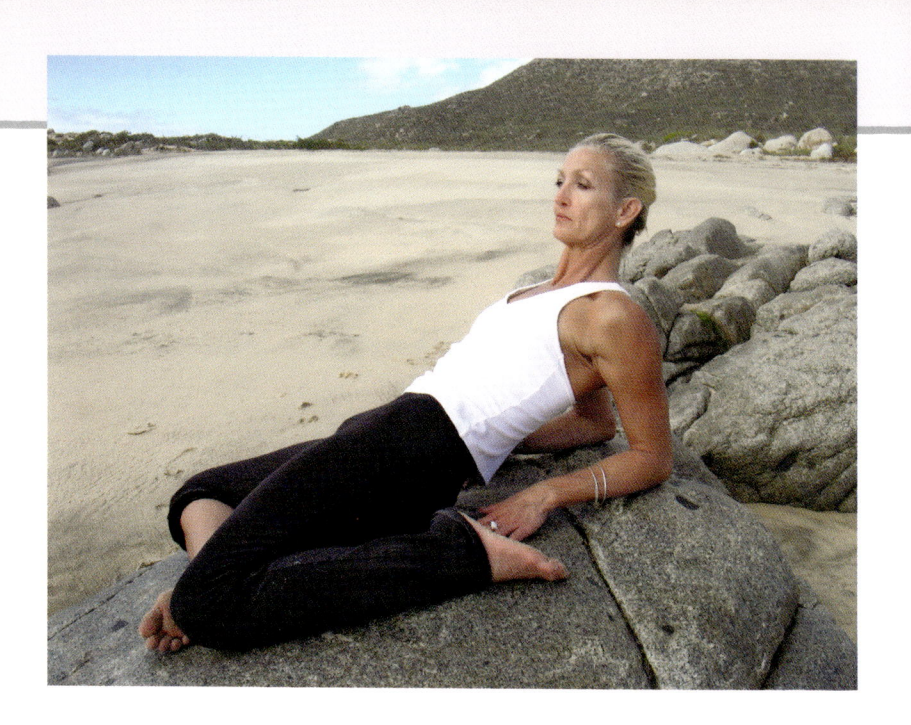

Quadriceps Stretch

Sit your butt down on the ground.

Press the inside of the left knee on the ground and the left heel toward the buttocks with the foot gently turned out away from your sitbones. The sole of the other foot can rest lightly against the left knee. The legs have a sort of pinwheel look. Lean back on your right elbow or hand. Look for a straight line from the left kneecap through the right shoulder. Pull the left hip back toward the floor as if to open the flat lower belly to the sky. It is really important to keep the knee of the leg which is experiencing the quadriceps stretch consistently on the ground.

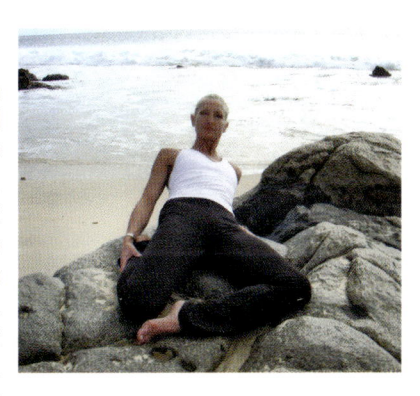

To intensify the stretch, gently squeeze the left buttock without tucking it under. Think of the length of the stretching leg spinning away from its hipbone (ASIS) like the spoke of a wheel turning. Inhale for a count of four and exhale for four counts and repeat three times.

Repeat with the right knee down and stretch the right quadriceps and hip flexor.

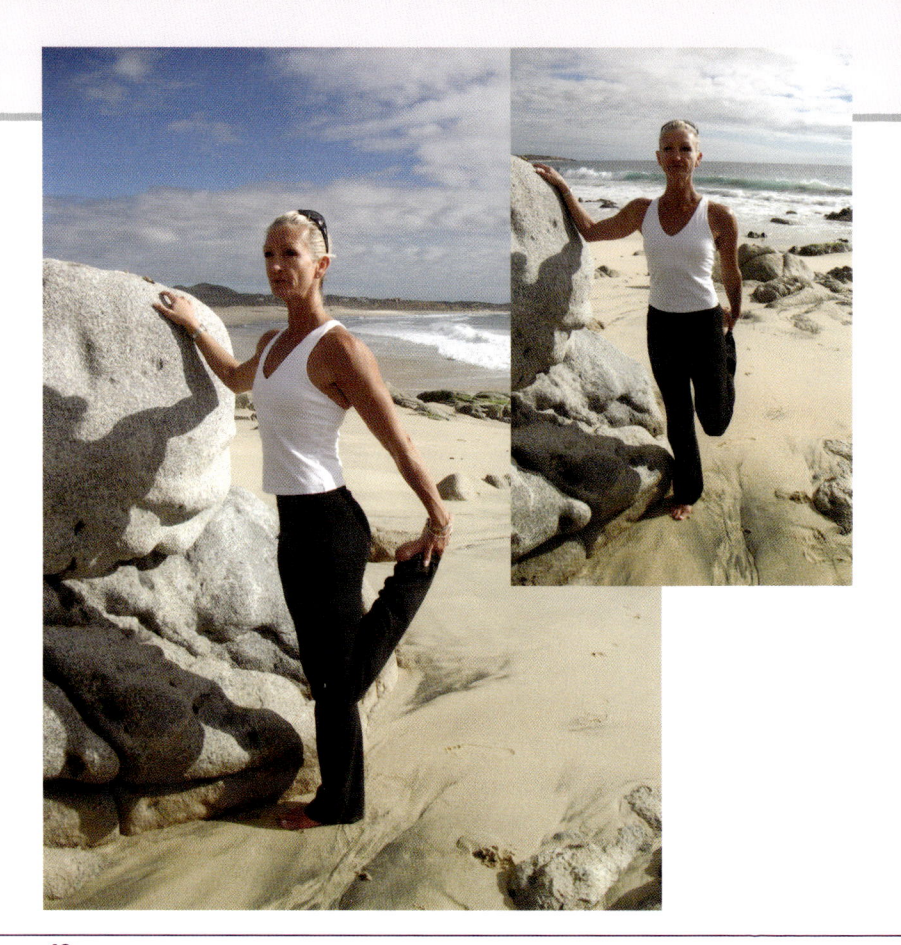

Standing Quadriceps Stretch

The great thing about the **Standing Quadriceps Stretch** is that you really can do it anywhere, standing in the interminable checkout line at the market, waiting at the bus stop, in the middle of your very long walk to decrease discomfort and increase your stamina. The downside, though, is that a lot of attention goes toward balance and knee safety. Balance practices are certainly not a bad thing, but neither the stretch nor the proprioceptive aspect are enhanced by being challenged at the same time.

If you do the **Standing Quadriceps Stretch,** stand first with both feet parallel (second toes and center of heels same distance apart) and legs parallel between the hipbones (ASIS) and the pubic bones. Bring one heel up toward the sitbone. Grasp the front of the foot with the hand on the same side of the body and gently press the foot into the hand. This protects the knee from overflexing. Then press the knee backward and gently pull with the hand. Be really sure the knee is under the hip, not out to the side of the hip. Hold something for balance, or focus your eyes softly on something that is not moving to improve balance while you stand on one leg.

Inhale for a count of four and exhale for a count of four and repeat the breathing cycle three times. Carefully release the foot to the ground. Notice the difference between the legs. Gently bend the other knee and pull the heel to the sitbone to stretch the other leg.

(If you are doing the full Practice, the Quadriceps Stretch in the seated position will flow into the next stretch, the Sides of Buttocks and Thighs. You do not have to also do the Standing Stretch.)

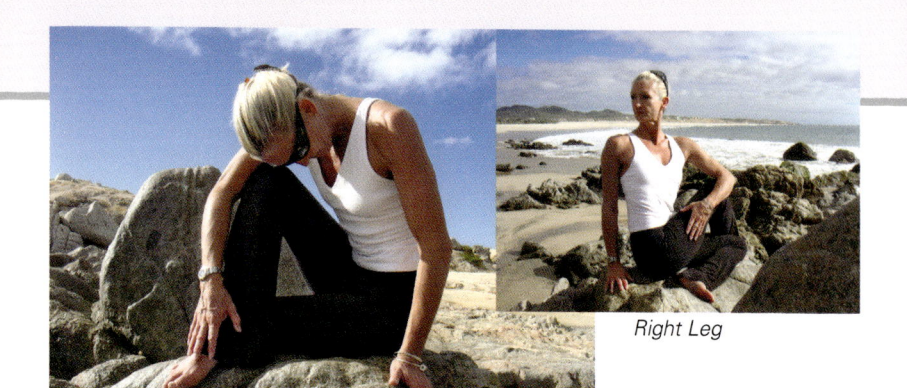

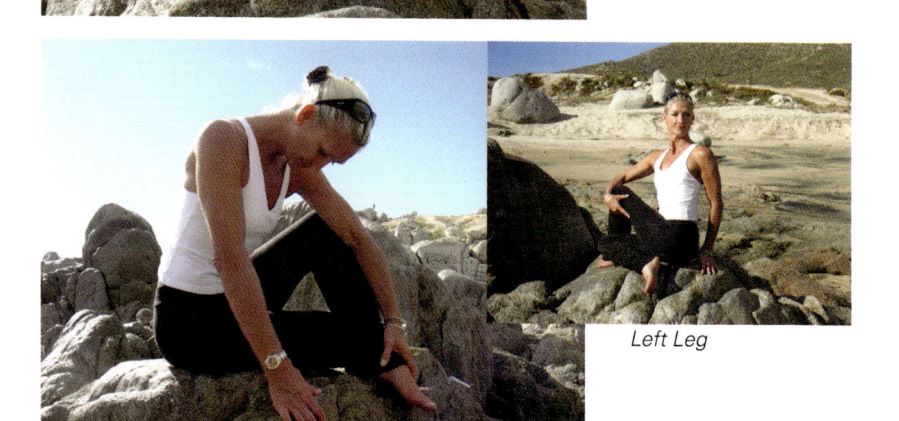

Right Leg

Left Leg

SIDES OF BUTTOCKS AND THIGHS

Do the **Quadriceps Stretch** before the sides of the hips. The **Sides of Buttocks and Thighs** is intended to target the buttocks muscles, the sides of the thighs, and maybe the iliotibial band for some people.

Sit on your sitbones. Bend the left knee so it points out in front of you and is centered with the pubic bones. The left foot will be by the right sitbone but don't sit on it. Bend the right knee upward and place the right heel in front of, or to the left of your left knee. Follow the line of your right shinbone with your right hand, and continue to trace the shin line with your forearm, in order to stretch your torso forward and on the diagonal to the left. Let the head hang. Keep the right sitbone on the ground. Wow. Breathe, eh?

Inhale for a count of four and exhale for four counts and repeat three times. Repeat with the right knee forward, left knee up and stretching torso and top of head toward the right. Notice which side is tighter. Be in this stretch a bit longer on the tight side.

Add spine rotation by sitting up straight and putting the left hand or elbow on the right knee and gently pulling to twist the spine to the right.

47 Wee Small Stretch Book

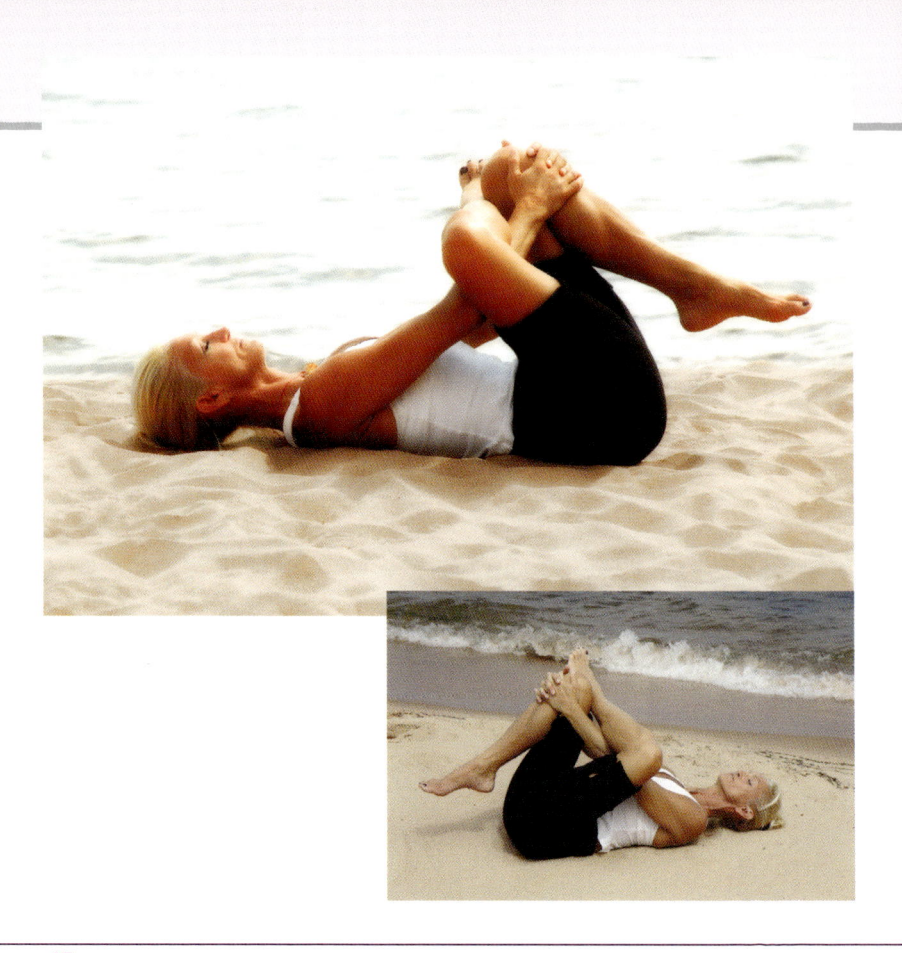

EXTERNAL ROTATORS STRETCH

The **External Rotators Stretch** is possibly less intense than the **Hurdle Stretch** in the **Quad/Hips/Hamstrings Series,** and you can be more specific about the location of the stretch.

From the **Sides of Buttocks and Thighs Stretch,** lie down on your back. Cross the right ankle over the left thighbone at the knee. Bring the left thighbone over the chest and hold close to the chest by wrapping the left arm around the leg and the right arm through the legs. Let the shoulders and arms feel heavy so they are not wrapped up around your ears. Allow your head to stay on the floor and let the neck feel free, relaxed. Align your hips and shoulders parallel with each other. Gently and continuously pull the left leg into the body. This is a great position to feel breathing into your backbones and back muscles. Feel your back spread out over the earth. Feel the release in the deep right buttock.

Inhale for a count of four and exhale for four counts and repeat three times. Release the legs. Place the left ankle over the right thighbone at the knee. Repeat. Intensify the stretch by pulling the sitbones down toward the earth.

49 Wee Small Stretch Book

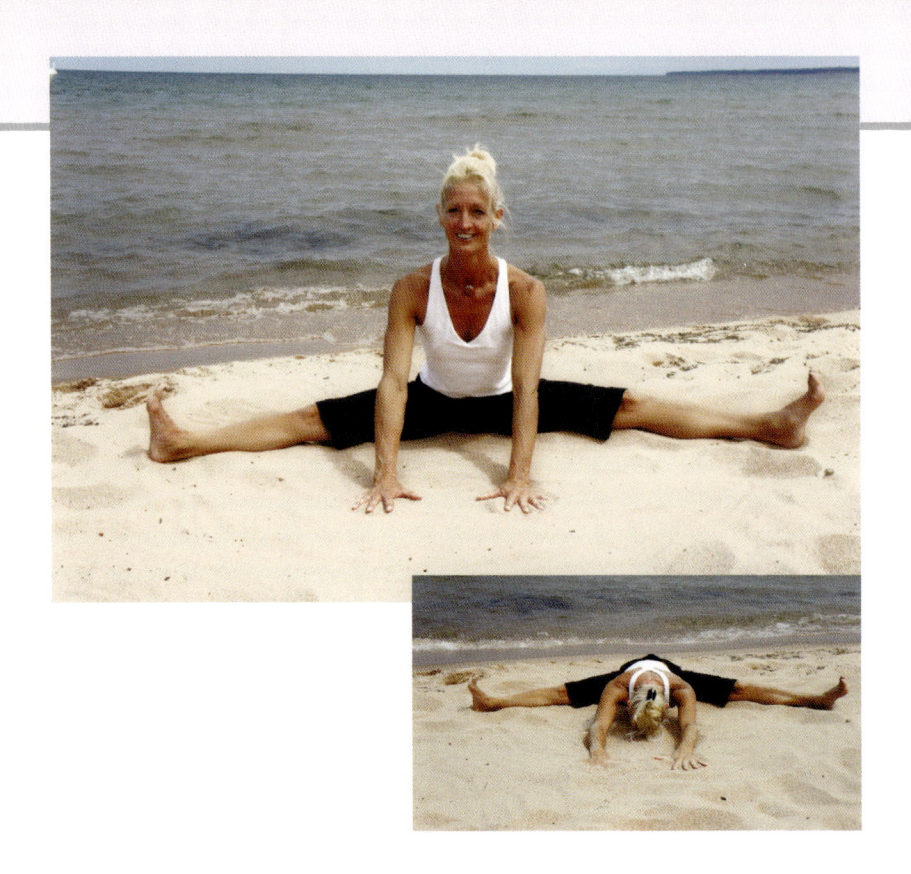

Inner Thigh Stretch

From the **External Rotators Stretch,** come up to sitting. Sit on your sitbones. If you do not have enough flexibility to be on your bones without rounding your back behind your sitbones, sit up on a block or rolled mat or towel or the curb. Place your feet wider than your pelvis, as wide as you can without strain. The toes should point straight up. Kneecaps should aim straight up. It is okay to bend the knees, but keep pulling the sitbones away from the feet. Do not let your knees roll in or out. Keep your back straight and your head on the end of your neck instead of in front of your body.

Pitch forward from the femoral joint, where your leg bones come into your pelvis, until your hands touch the floor. Breathe. Wait for the inner thigh muscles to release. Walk your hands forward, keeping your back straight up the spine and flat across the back width. Inhale for a count of four and exhale for four counts and repeat three times. Think of your legs feeling heavy. Think of your body falling softly forward. Feel the leg bones run like mercury off the ends of the earth.

51 Wee Small Stretch Book

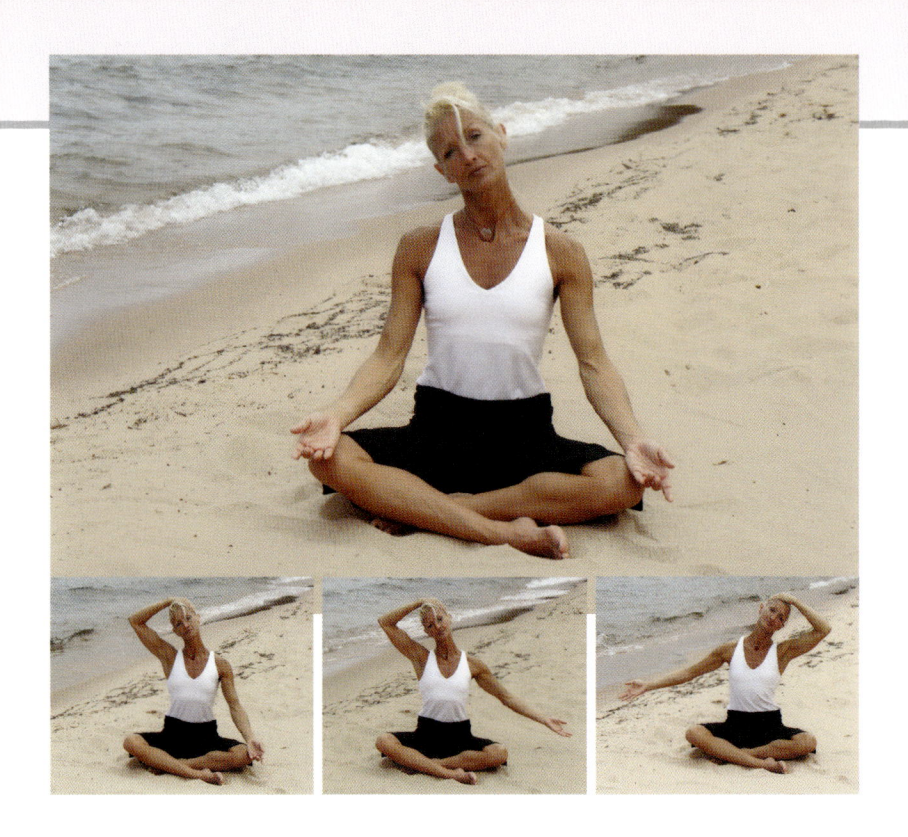

Neck Stretch

Neck Front

To stretch the left front of your neck, hold the left pectoral chest muscle with left hand on top of breast. Cover the left hand with the right hand. Hold the muscles into the ribs and down. Then lift the chin up and slightly to the right. Do not jam down the back of your neck. Breathe. Inhale for four counts and exhale for four counts and repeat three times. Stretch the right front of the neck. (There is no picture for this.)

Neck Side

To stretch the sides of the neck, look straight ahead. Pull your earlobes back and the points of your ears up. Let your right ear tip sideways to the right shoulder. You should still be looking straight ahead, not down or up. Return to vertical. Place your right hand on the upper left skull. Do not pull. Press your head into the hand gently. Guide your skull to the right shoulder with the right hand, then return neck to vertical by pressing the skull *into* the hand. Repeat four times. Inhale toward the shoulder, exhale toward vertical. Take your hand off of your skull before you let it return to vertical the last time - notice the "float" feeling.

For more intense stretch, reach the opposite arm on a diagonal line away from the body. Be really gentle. The neck stretch is a strong feeling to begin with since it is done so seldom. The neck stretch can be done standing or sitting. Just be sure the torso is stacked on top of the pelvis and not in front of it as you think about what you look like from the side. DO NOT twist or rotate your head or neck while stretching.

Stretch the other side of the neck.

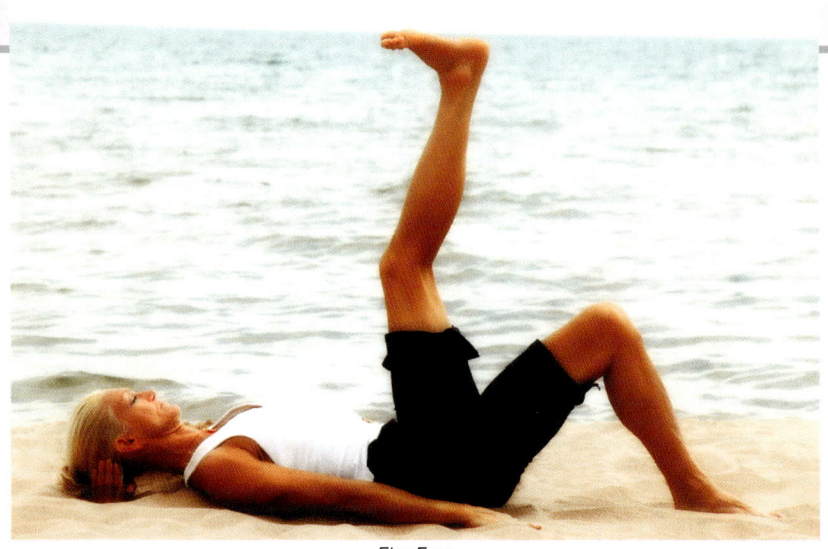

Flat Foot

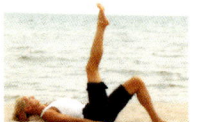

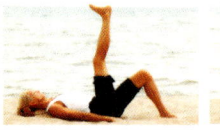

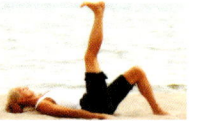

Plantar Flex High Heel   Plantar Flex Toes Ballet   Dorsiflex Ankle Dome   Dorsiflex Toes Elf

Foot/Ankle

Foot/Ankle (dorsi and plantar flexion of ankle and toes)

Lift your right leg in the air, keeping the knee slightly flexed. Foot flat to the ceiling or sky is the start position.

- Plantar Flex your ankle - the foot looks like it could be wearing a high heel shoe
- Plantar Flex your toes - the foot looks like it could be wearing a ballet pointe shoe
- Dorsiflex the ankle – the top of the foot has a dome shape toward the body
- Dorsiflex the toes – the foot looks like elf shoes

Repeat sequence three times, moving the foot as if carving through clay. Synchronize your breathing so that you inhale or exhale each time you change position in the ankle or toes. Breathe to move.

Reverse the order:

- Plantar Flex the toes – dome foot
- Plantar Flex the ankle - ballet foot
- Dorsiflex the toes – high heel foot
- Dorsiflex the ankles – elf foot

Circle the foot three times each direction. Repeat with other foot.

55 Wee Small Stretch Book

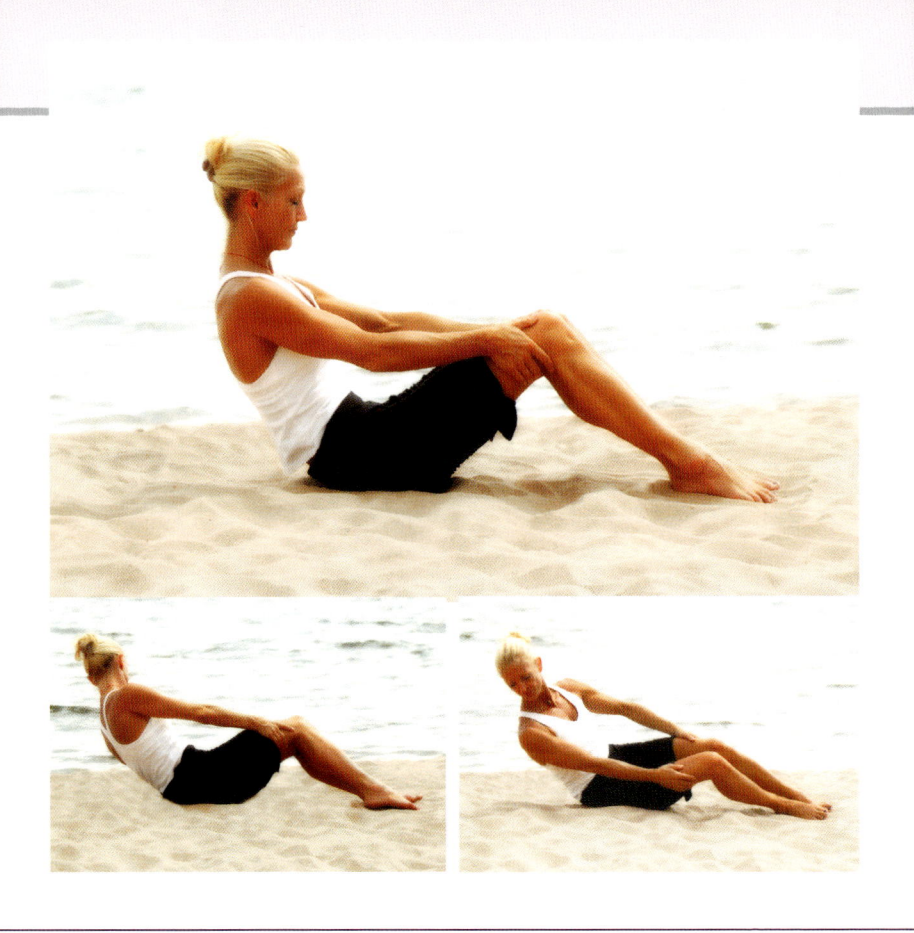

Abdominal Curls

An incredibly efficient abdominal conditioning effort, the abdominal curls will stretch your back and strengthen your exhale muscles. Sit behind your sitbones, knees bent up to the sky, legs pressed tightly together. Cross your forearms over your lower belly wall. Curve the entire spine but don't let the head hang or be pulled forward. Inhale as you roll one vertebra at a time back toward the floor. Keep the abdominals from bulging out. Exhale, reverse direction by lifting one vertebra at a time away from the floor, bringing torso back toward the thighbones. Curl the tailbone toward the forehead. Stay in your belly. Stay out of your hip flexors. Repeat three times.

Sit on your right buttock, tipping to the right, look over your right shoulder toward the floor. Inhale to curl the side of the spine down toward the floor; exhale to curl back up. Think of being a shrimp. Repeat three times and then shift to the left buttock and repeat three.

Whew. Pretty efficient to get all your ab work done in 9 moves and improve your breathing too. If this is too challenging to begin with, place hands on the back of the hamstrings and support the torso in the curls.

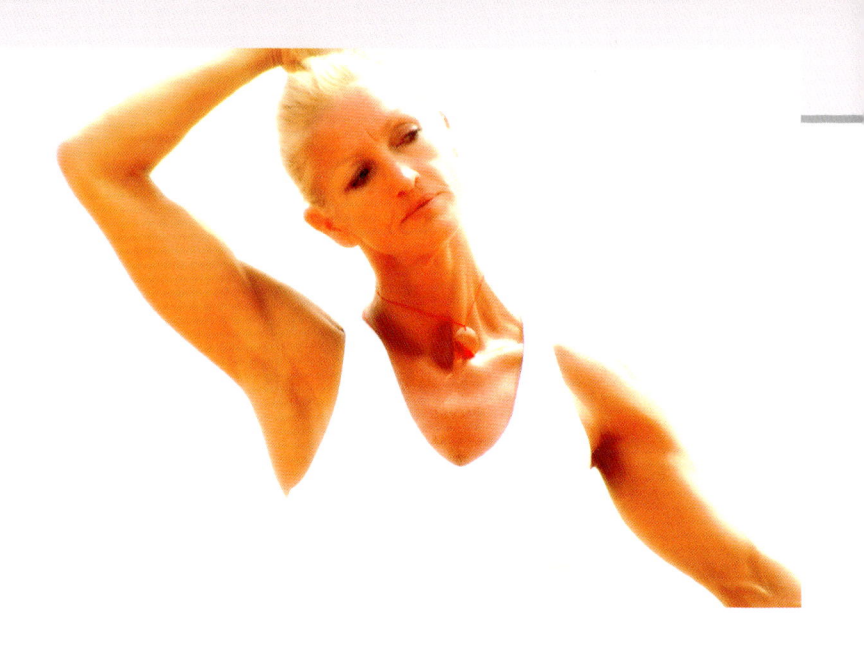

Can Do Today

If you cannot take the time for the full practice, take 10 minutes every day.

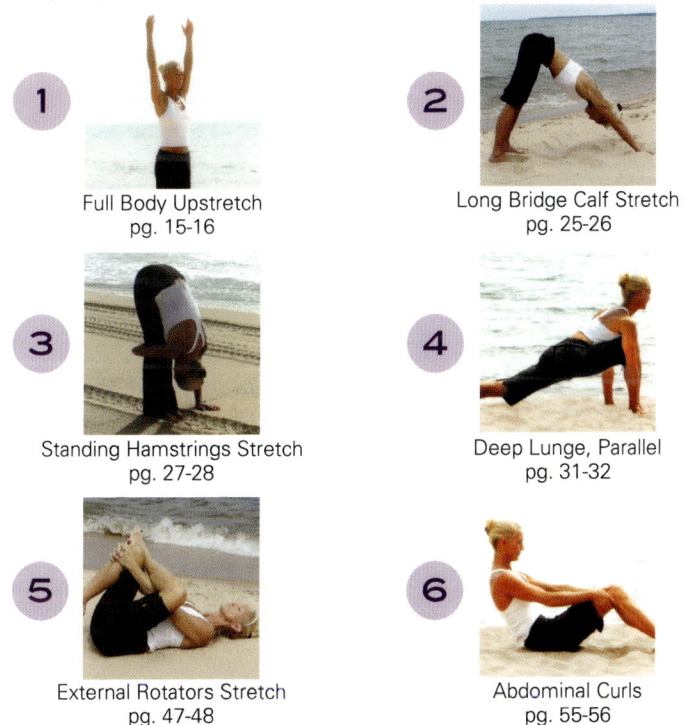

1. Full Body Upstretch
pg. 15-16

2. Long Bridge Calf Stretch
pg. 25-26

3. Standing Hamstrings Stretch
pg. 27-28

4. Deep Lunge, Parallel
pg. 31-32

5. External Rotators Stretch
pg. 47-48

6. Abdominal Curls
pg. 55-56

The Full Practice in Pictures

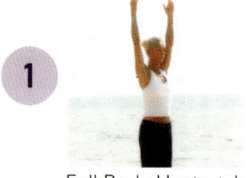

1 Full Body Upstretch
pg. 15-16

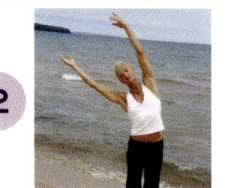

2 Torso Side Stretch
pg. 17-18

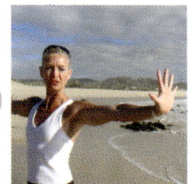

3 Jazz Hands and Arms Stretch
pg. 19-20

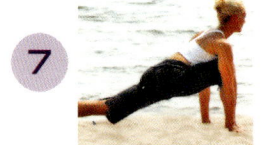

7 Deep Lunge, Parallel
pg. 31-32

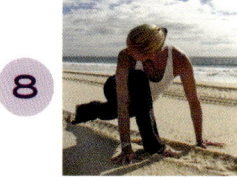

8 Deep Lunge, Rotated
pg. 33-34

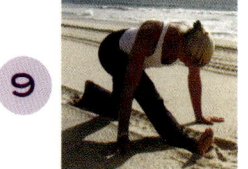

9 Hamstrings, Parallel
pg. 35-36

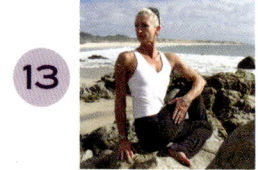

13 Sides of Buttocks and Thighs
pg. 45-46

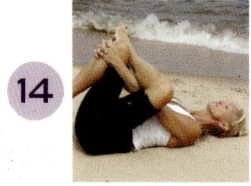

14 External Rotators Stretch
pg. 47-48

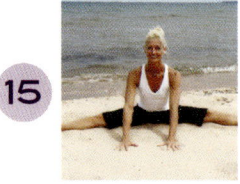

15 Inner Thigh Stretch
pg. 49-50

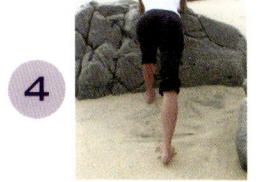

4 Standing Calf Stretch
pg. 23-24

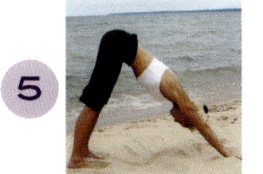

5 Long Bridge Calf Stretch
pg. 25-26

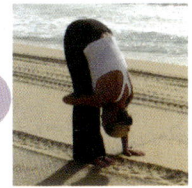

6 Standing Hamstrings Stretch
pg. 27-28

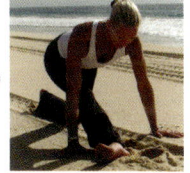

10 Hamstrings, Rotated
pg. 37-38

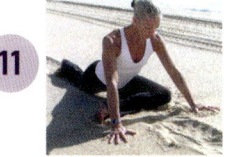

11 Hurdle Stretch
pg. 39-40

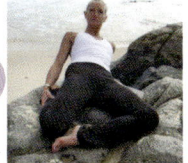

12 Quadriceps Stretch
pg. 41-42

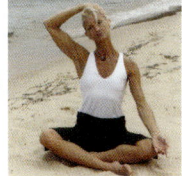

16 Neck Stretch
pg. 51-52

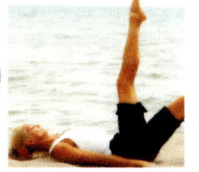

17 Foot/Ankle
pg. 53-54

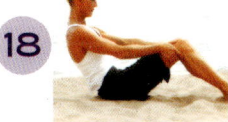

18 Abdominal Curls
pg. 55-56

BIOGRAPHY

In the late 90's, Kathleen Conklin transitioned from a career in law to teaching stretch and strength techniques, and the Pilates Method of Physical and Mental Conditioning. She continues to explore the vast shimmering depth of this cognitive movement work.

- Stretch and Strength class teacher, PilateSpa, Body Conscious, LLC, and Gold's Gym, 1998 - present
- Author of chapters on "Breathing" and "Stretching" for 'CycleOps Pro 300 PT' Manual, for Saris Cycling Group
- UW-Madison, Dissection Anatomy, 1989
- UW-Madison, Dance Department, 1980-1984, studies with Judy Alter, author of <u>Stretch & Strengthen</u>
- Madeline Black Pilates, CA
- Michael Miller Pilates, Boulder, CO
- The Pilates Center, Boulder, CO
- Pilates Studio of the Midwest in Evanston, IL 1998, teacher training

Kathleen Conklin owns Body Conscious, LLC, operating PilateSpa, Madison, WI.

www.PilateSpa.com